Home Remedies

EXPRESS

Home Remedies Express

Home Remedies

EXPRESS

Know How to Cure the Most Common
Health Issues Using Natural Home
Remedies

Katherine Kelley & KnowIt Express

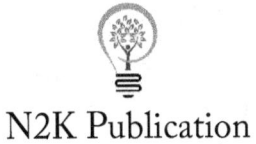

N2K Publication

ISBN 978-1-533-00418-5

Printed in the United States of America

First Edition

Welcome to the *Know It Express* - the express lane to knowledge!

To stay up-to-date, please be sure to sign up for **our newsletter** at http://www.KnowItExpress.com and follow us on social media:

https://www.facebook.com/KnowItExpress
https://twitter.com/KnowItExpress
https://plus.google.com/+KnowItExpress

EXPRESS LANE

Home Remedies Express

CHAPTER 1

Using Home Remedies to Improve Your Health

Ancient World Cures

Diseases and ill-health are some of life's miseries and, unfortunately, we cannot predict with certainty when they will occur. Some illnesses can become worse if not treated immediately. Thankfully, our great ancestors have provided us with solutions to some of life's less serious afflictions.

Home remedies have a place in history.

Thinking back to the time before modern medicine played the role it does today, how did people resolve their illnesses? That's right, **home remedies**. And people still use many of them today.

Think about the times you have had a nice hot bowl of *Campbell's Chicken Noodle Soup* when you feel a cold coming on. Or the honey you add to your tea when your throat hurts. Has your mother ever said "Grandma used to (insert Grandma's solution here) for that" or said "This remedy has been in our family for years!" Those are examples of remedies used by our ancestors.

OR maybe you've found yourself sick in the middle of the night when all the pharmacies within a 10 miles radius of you are closed or you are in an unfamiliar location where the closest health center is miles away? It feels like you're in a bad movie plot when that happens. **Relief.** You just want relief. **Now.**

Bringing Back Old Practices

This is where home remedies can come in most handy; they can start to give relief within minutes. Home remedies are hands-on *on hand* relief that you can get without having to leave the house.

Home remedies, in the simplest explanation, are the use of herbs, spices, and other foods or plants to cure *common* health ailments. Isn't that simple enough? What's more, these can be sourced commercially or grown in the backyard

So yes, home remedy does have a place in modern society. But as a <u>disclaimer</u>: always seek help from professional medical health providers first before attempting any holistic approach. Homeopathy should only act as secondary options if appropriate situations arise.

CHAPTER 2

Some Common Health Ailments to Know

There are many health challenges you or others are bound to see on a fairly frequent basis. They can be serious or trivial, and their causes and symptoms vary (although symptoms often overlap between illnesses). Some of them include:

Common Health Ailment 1: Diarrhea

Diarrhea causes loss of high amounts of fluid through persistent passing of watery stool caused by various conditions or situations such as:

- Gastroenteritis.
- Irritable Bowel Syndrome.
- Poor diet.
- Consumption of laxatives.

Common Health Ailment 2: Acid Reflux

Anyone in their 40's may remember this 80's commercial: "How do *you* spell relief?" Cut to answer: "R-O-L-A-I-D-S." Rolaids help acid reflux, which is the upward movement of fluids from the stomach to the esophagus. In the process, gastric acid, made up in part of diluted hydrochloric acid (HCL), goes up with the fluid and erodes the delicate lining of the esophagus resulting in:

- Heartburn.
- Halitosis (bad breath).
- Burning feeling in the throat from the acid.

Common Health Ailment 3: Body Odor

Have you ever hugged someone or come close to a friend and then noticed an odor impossible to ignore? That is probably body odor. Body odor can be a sign of:

- Poor personal hygiene (not showering for days by choice, for example).
- Hyperhidrosis, a medical condition in which people suffer from excessive sweating.
- Stress.

Common Health Ailment 4: Constipation

Constipation causes difficulty in passing stool as one normally would. Causes of constipation may be:

- Poor diet.
- Medications.
- Medical Conditions.

Common Health Ailment 5: Headache

Headache is that throbbing pain that occurs anywhere in your head. If you're one of the very limited population to never have had a headache, you are lucky as they can range from dull and bothersome, such as a simple headache with a cold, to very debilitating, such as a migraine where some require a completely black room to help resolve it because any kind of light accentuates the pain. Some common causes are:

- Stress.
- Poor Air Quality.
- Foods.

Common Health Ailment 6: Insomnia

Insomnia is the medical term used when you have difficulty in sleeping or you cannot sleep for long periods of time. Insomnia can be acute or chronic, and is caused by:

- Stress.

- Medications.
- Depression.

Common Health Ailment 7: Common Cold

A cold is a viral infection in a person's upper respiratory system. You know what happens: the weather becomes frigid, your nose starts running, you start looking like Rudolph the Red-nosed Reindeer after blowing your nose for what seems like the 100th time in 4 hours, your throat hurts because your glands swell, and no amount of Campbell's Chicken Noodle Soup will get rid of your chills. You feel just *miserable*, like you could be the spokesperson for Nyquil, Halls, *and* Puffs Plus w/ Lotion. More general common causes can be:

- Extreme weather changes within short periods of time.
- Viral Infection from touching improperly washed surfaces.
- Not dressing appropriately for the weather.

Common Health Ailment 8: Fever

Fever is the rise in temperature beyond *your* "normal" temperature, whatever that may be. Fever often comes with headache and shivering and, if too high (in excess of 103 degrees Fahrenheit), febrile convulsions, disorientation, or dehydration may result. Causes include:

- Hypothermia (remember Buffalo, NY getting 7 *feet* of snow in 2014?).
- Influenza.
- Internal physical issues.

Common Health Ailment 9: Fatigue

This, in the simplest definition, is the inability to function due to depletion of necessary abilities to perform the functions. Fatigue comes in two variations: physical and mental. Physical fatigue is the inability of muscles to expend enough energy to exert force because cellular waste product accumulates faster than it is removed. Mental fatigue is the inability to think clearly due to prolonged periods of cognitive engagement. Causes of both variations include:

- Stress.
- Lack of proper and *quality* sleep.
- Poor diet.

Common Health Ailment 10: Indigestion

Indigestion happens when the food you take in is not broken down and absorbed properly. This will result in pain in the abdomen. This may cause pain, heartburn, or a feeling of uncomfortable fullness. Causes:

- Poor Diet.
- Eating too fast.
- Medical Conditions.

Common Health Ailment 11: Food Poisoning

Maybe you have had the experience where you consumed a meal but came down with diarrhea, vomiting or nausea within an hour or two of eating. Causes of food poisoning include eating:

- Undercooked meats.
- Expired foods.
- Foods with (often unintentionally) harmful chemicals or preservatives.

Common Health Ailment 12: Inflammation

Inflammation can occur when any part of the body sustains blunt force trauma such as a broken arm from a fall off a bike, to a simpler example of an insect bite or sting. However, blunt force is not the only cause of inflammation; there are plenty that can result *without* any type of blunt force, bite, or sting. Some of those causes include:

- Appendicitis (inflammation of the appendix).

- Gastroenteritis (infection within the stomach lining).
- Sinusitis (inflammation of space within the nose).

Common Health Ailment 13: Dandruff And Scalp Irritation

Dandruff is a fungal attack on the scalp making your head itch causing white flakes often seen by others on your shoulders. Dandruff sufferers are often embarrassed by all the flakes seen. Causes of dandruff include:

- Insufficient and/or infrequent shampooing of your hair.
- Eczema.
- Contact dermatitis.

Common Health Ailment 14: Tooth Discoloration/Tooth Enamel Erosion

Depending on your diet and age, your teeth may become discolored. It is normal that enamel wears off the more we use our teeth, but there are causes that accelerate the discoloration and loss of enamel such as:

- Coffee.
- Smoking.
- Poor dental hygiene.

Common Health Ailment 15: Back And Joint Pain

Sometimes you may want to lift something heavy from the ground and instead of the object going up, you end up going down with a pain on your lower back. Causes of back pain include:

- Improper lifting techniques.
- Insufficient exercise.
- Excessive body weight.

*****

While this list seems exhaustive, there are still hundreds of common health challenges. This list will, at the very least, help you understand the broad nature of ailments in which home remedies can be applied.

CHAPTER 3

Getting Started with Home Remedies

Different Types Of Components

No one becomes knowledgeable in any topic without practicing. The first step to getting started with home remedy is learning about different ingredients and how they work as remedies.

Ingredients to home remedies can be found at supermarkets, farmers markets, health food stores, and even "big-box" stores. So, what *are* some of the "right" items?

1) **Fruits & Vegetables.** Fruits and vegetables have different colors, firmness, sizes, and scents when ripe; be sure to choose carefully. For more information, go to http://efed.aces.illinois.edu/eaters/Images/FV%20in%20Season.pdf.

2) **Herbs & Spices.** Herbs and spices have a wide variety of benefits. For more in-depth information, we recommend you peruse http://usesofherbs.com.

3) **Grains, Nuts, Seeds.** These items, as with both of the above, have various benefits, and can usually be eaten by themselves or as part of meal. A good starting point for more information about these can be found at http://www.ironman.com/triathlon-news/articles/2012/12/the-importance-of-seeds-and-grains.aspx#axzz3x5nQpGTp.

Where To Get Ingredients

There are also online stores from where you can order your home remedies and health supplements, but of course you can always go to your local health food and herbal shops.

A few examples are:

1) Bulk Herb Store (http://www.bulkherbstore.com): They have a good selection of dried herbs from which you can select. Their YouTube channel also has helpful video tutorials; simply click on the video link on the far right hand side of the home page for several "how to" videos available for download.

2) Mountain Rose Herbs (https://www.mountainroseherbs.com): Their selection of dried herbs is excellent. In addition, this site has a number of books available for purchase ranging from body care to plant identification. Simply click on the "Home Goods" tab at the top of the page, and then click on "Books and Education" at the far left of the following page.

3) Vitacost (http://www.vitacost.com): This is a great site for low cost dried herbs. They offer a discount for first time customers, and have other helpful resources such as recipes for eating clean.

Maintain Best Practices

Best practices are standards met and actions done repeatedly and consistently because they have proven efficacy. In regards to foods included in home remedies, "best practices" are the following:

1) Washing all fruits and vegetables prior to cutting or eating.

2) Cutting everything into required proportions to aid in digestion.

3) Using fresh and ripe foods.

<u>Exercise</u>: Flashcards Aren't Just For Children

As stated, part of learning is repetition and practice. Sometimes the best way to do this is to use old school methods. So, let's create some flashcards.

1) Buy at least 35 index cards, or make index cards by cutting pieces of paper into 35 equal size squares.

2) Make 35 flashcards using five of each of the following: fruits, vegetables, herbs, spices, nuts, grains, and seeds.

3) Label the front of each card with the name of each of the foods.

4) Label the back of the card with one health benefit and an ailment for which you would use it.

5) When cards have been completed, begin quizzing yourself.

6) As you memorize each of the cards, remove it to continue working on those which you don't know as well.

7) When you get to zero, quiz yourself on them again.

8) After the second round, create more flashcards with new foods and repeat the process.

CHAPTER 4

Natural Remedies for Common Health Ailments

In the previous sections you have learned about home remedies and some of the common health challenges. Now is the time to put all you have learned into practice. For each of the following diseases, prepare a home remedy to cure the ailment as follows:

Natural Ailment Remedy 1: Diarrhea

Diarrhea causes loss of fluid and ions such as potassium and sodium which you will need to replace. The best way to do that is using one of the two following solutions:

A) Oral Rehydration Therapy (ORT). Prepare ORT in the following way:

- Get 1 Tbsp. of salt, 2 Tbsp. of granulated sugar, and 16 fl. Oz. of clean water.

- Pour the salt and sugar into the water and shake to dissolve.

- Heat the water up to 104 degrees Fahrenheit to make sure the solutes dissolves completely.

- Drink intermittently to make up for the loss of water until the diarrhea stops.

B) Yogurt. Yogurt, in general, is very good for preventing diarrhea that may be caused by bacteria in food. It contains probiotics, which are "good" bacteria added to foods in order to help attack the bad bacteria often found in diarrhea.

And chances are you're familiar with Jamie Lee Curtis and her *Activia Challenge* (and its jingle that is now stuck in your head). Well, it's not just for women who are getting older and experiencing changes in their digestive processes. It's for anyone who needs it.

In addition to yogurt, foods that contain probiotics are:

- Cheeses such as Gouda, Parmesan or cottage cheeses.

- Fermented vegetables such as pickles.

- Dark chocolate (and who doesn't want an excuse to eat dark chocolate).

- Sauerkraut.

Natural Ailment Remedy 2: Acid Reflux

Acid reflux causes a lot of discomfort and a burning sensation where your stomach and lower esophagus meet so you will need a remedy to neutralize or absorb the acid. Remedies for combating Acid Reflux are:

A) Ginger Root

- Can be purchased at most grocery stores. It is generally found in the fresh fruits and vegetables section.

- Intake of Ginger should be strictly limited to no more than 4g per day. This would include Ginger in liquids and foods.

- Choose young ginger roots as they contain more juice than their more mature counterparts.

- Grate ginger root on to foods, or use to make tea. Recipes can be found online.

B) Fennel

- Has the ability to reduce spasm of stomach walls (because of a compound in it called Anethole) which prevents vomiting.

- Can be bought in seed or vegetable form to add to recipes.

- Can reduce gas and bloating in addition to acid reflux.

Natural Ailment Remedy 3: Body Odor

Fighting body odor has to do with getting rid of the odor causing bacteria, which are predominantly found in the armpit because there is reduced opportunity for your arm pits to "breathe" and thus stay dry. Controlling body odor can be done in the following ways:

A) Wiping the armpit with a cotton ball soaked in alcohol.

B) Taking multiple showers in a day if necessary and washing armpits thoroughly.

C) Wearing clothes that "breathe" as some fabrics, such as polyester, retain body odor.

Natural Ailment Remedy 4: Constipation

Constipation can be treated by increasing bowel movement. You can achieve this by:

A) Taking two tablespoons of olive oil or flax seed oil before eating your meals. This will coat the intestine to enhance bowel movement.

B) Increasing your water intake.

C) Going on a fruit fast.

- Get assorted fruits e.g. apples, oranges, lemon, banana etc. (anything from the citrus family is most preferable because of the fibrous inside) Wash the fruits and cut them into smaller bits.

- Mix them and serve with a glass of milk.

- Substitute this for your morning breakfast.

Natural Ailment Remedy 5: Headache

Remedies for curing headaches are fairly simple. They include:

A) Exercise regularly.

B) Get sufficient sleep that includes REM (Rapid Eye Movement) sleep.

C) Give yourself a steam bath with Rosemary by doing the following:

- Harvest a few handfuls of the herb.

- Place in a liter of water in a pot and heat until it steams.

- Pour the steaming liquid plus the herbs into a big bowl.

- Grab a large towel and place it over your head.

- Bend over the bowl, keeping your face at least 6 inches from the boiling water, and place the towel over the entire bowl to trap the steam.

- Inhale the steam from the mixture for one to two minutes.

Natural Ailment Remedy 6: Insomnia

To relieve yourself of insomnia, you need to slow your brain and your body down. This can be done in one of the following ways:

A) Drink warm milk immediately prior to bed.

- Pour 8 to 12 oz. of milk in a pot.

- Heat milk for approximately 8-10 minutes, or until warm.

- Let cool slightly if too hot; drink when tolerable.

- The warmth will slightly increase your body temperature, calming your nerves, making you feel sleepy.

B) Limit caffeine intake. While it's not required to cut yourself off completely from caffeine, it is best to stop drinking caffeinated products well before bed (in the early afternoon, for example) so that it has an opportunity to work itself out of your system in time for bed.

C) Create a nightly routine. Parents do it with children, but it's just important for adults to do if for themselves. An example of a routine would be:

- Turn TV off at 8:00 P.M.

- Read in bed for only 30 minutes.

- Brush teeth and wash face at 9:00 P.M.

- Turn lights out by 9:15 P.M.

Natural Ailment Remedy 7: Common Cold

Chances are you have a go-to remedy for the common cold, but if you don't, here are a couple for you:

A) Garlic, Ginger, & Honey Mixture

- Get one fairly large root of ginger and peel off the skin.

- Get two cloves of garlic and peel off the white flaky skin.

- Put the garlic and the ginger into a blender and add about 4 fl. Oz. of clean water.

- Blend until smooth.

- Strain the blend and add the liquid to half a liter of natural honey.

- Take two Tbsp. every morning and night for seven days. If your bout of the flu is severe, take more frequently.

- If your cold hasn't resolved after seven days, seek medical attention.

B) Add spices such as Cumin or Turmeric to food; these will aid in heating up your body, pushing toxins out.

C) Take a steam shower. Steam will cause mucus to break up and drain out of your body.

Natural Ailment Remedy 8: Fever

When your body temperature begins to rise and subsequently stay at a temperature higher than your normal average body temperature, you have a fever. Ways to bring down your fever include:

A) Taking a *lukewarm* shower.

B) Covering yourself under 3 or 4 blankets to "break" the fever by "sweating it out."

C) Putting a cool washcloth on your forehead or neck.

Natural Ailment Remedy 9: Fatigue

Fatigue can be handled by inducing alertness. One can accomplish this by doing the following:

A) Add 2 grams of coffee to your tea.

B) Add diffuser reeds to an open bottle of peppermint or eucalyptus oil. Reeds can be purchased online or at stores like Bed, Bath & Beyond.

C) Maintain a healthy and balanced diet. High amounts of "junk food" in your daily diet will tend to make you sleepy.

Natural Ailment Remedy 10: Indigestion

According to the Mayo Clinic, some of the best natural remedies for indigestion are:

A) Getting enough sleep to help reduce stress.

B) Exercise regularly and maintain a healthy weight.

C) Eat smaller and more frequent meals, and include foods rich in fiber such as bananas, pears, and almonds to name a few examples.

- A comprehensive list can be found by going to MayoClinic.org and enter in "high fiber food chart" in the search engine for the site. A link will be provided that will take you to the chart (it should be first on the list that populates after searching the Mayo site).

Natural Ailment Remedy 11: Food Poisoning

While food poisoning typically takes care of itself in due time (normally within 24-48 hours), some people like to help the process along. Examples of home remedies for food poisoning include:

A) Lemon. Lemon is a very good anti-poison because its acid contents helps to kill off the microbes causing the poisoning. To prepare lemon juice do the following:

- Get 5 ripe lemons.

- Peel and cut into two halves.

- Remove any seeds.

- Squeeze out the juice into a glass.

- Filter to get rid of the pulps.

- Add sugar (optional) for taste.

B) Have some clear broth.

C) Suck on ice chips.

Natural Ailment Remedy 12: Inflammation And Cuts

Inflammation is an ailment with a plethora of home remedies. Some examples include:

A) Cryotherapy. Ice brings down the swelling of the affected blood vessels in the area injured. Reduction in temperature will reduce the rate of blood flow, and subsequently, the swelling.

B) Herbs and Spices. Cumin, Turmeric and Rosemary are examples that help reduce swelling because of their anti-inflammatory properties.

C) Honey. Apply honey over the surface of an opened wound. *According to the *Department of Biological Sciences*, University of Waikato, Hamilton, New Zealand, honey acts as an effective wound dressing that promotes healing. The high sugar content of honey will induce coagulation of blood. Also, honey has antibacterial properties that, because of its high sugar content, organisms find it hard to survive on them. It's not surprising, then, why honey can store for years without getting spoiled.

*(http://www.ncbi.nlm.nih.gov/pubmed/16543212)

Natural Ailment Remedy 13: Dandruff And Scalp Irritation

Dandruff can be itchy and discomforting and is usually as a result of fungal infection. This can be curbed in the following ways:

A) Using Neem, a tree that has antibacterial properties. In order to prepare this remedy, do the following:

- Get a good quantity of neem leaves.

- Boil them until the water begins to green.

- Let the water cool to a tolerable, yet warm to hot temperature.

- Strain and use the fluid to wash your hair.

B) Apply apple cider vinegar (ACV) treatment.

- Combine equal parts water and ACV; a cup of each should do.

- Pour on hair and massage in as you would with shampoo.

- Massage into scalp for several minutes.

- Rinse treatment out of your hair.

- Do NOT shower immediately. Wait at least twelve hours before showering in order to give the treatment an opportunity to work.

- Repeat until fungal dandruff resolves.

C) Baking Soda.

- Take 1 Tbsp. of baking soda and mix it with 1 cup of water.

- Rub mixture into your scalp making sure to actually get down to the scalp. This will help in exfoliating the dead skin cells on your scalp.

- Rinse.

- Repeat as necessary.

Natural Ailment Remedy 14: Teeth Discoloration/Tooth Enamel Loss

Your diet and oral hygiene (or lack thereof) may cause your enamel to begin to turn yellow. Smokers also increase their risk of having yellowed teeth due to the tobacco content in cigarettes. To make your teeth as white as new, use the following remedies:

A) Baking soda. Baking soda acts like a bleach on your teeth. In addition to whitening your teeth, research has shown that sodium is a good antimicrobial and would help kill off harmful microbes in the mouth.

- Get few tablespoons of baking soda.

- Add lemon juice in drops and keep mixing until you have a paste.

- Apply the paste on your teeth and allow to stand for 2 to 3 minutes.

- Rinse.

- Repeat several times a week.

B) Lemon. The acidity of a lemon helps break down stains and return teeth to a whiter state. To use this as a home remedy, simply do the following:

- Cut a lemon in half.

- Rub the pulp of the lemon directly on your teeth for one minute.

- Rinse with lukewarm water.

C) Avoidance. Avoid food or drinks with deep, dark pigments, such as red wine or purple grape juice.

Natural Ailment Remedy 15: Back And Joint Pain

The spine, and body overall, is designed for movement. To accommodate this, it is made up of 23 vertebral discs and numerous major joints (think knee, elbow, shoulder, etc.). The following remedies will assist in reducing your pain:

A) Aerobic exercises, such as running, swimming, and cycling.

B) Cryotherapy, which can help reduce or resolve pain if used within the first few hours of onset.

C) Rest (for 48 hours). This doesn't mean to stay bedridden during that time, but rather don't overdo anything. After that time, work your way back to regular activity.

******

Now that you know what some remedies are, it's time to discuss how they can be applied.

CHAPTER 5

Application of Home Remedies

When To Use Home Remedies

We have gone over causes of some ailments and their remedies, but *when* do you actually use them?

The **best** time to use home remedies is the moment you begin to have slight symptoms of the ailment. If an illness gets too far out of control, it may end up requiring a more aggressive approach starting with a visit to a doctor.

If you've tried using a home remedy for 7 days and you have not seen significant improvement, it is advised that you seek medical attention.

Now, let's try some remedies.

Exercise: Know The Taste Of Your Own Medicine

Being proactive with regard to your health is important. No one wants to actually be sick while at the same time trying to figure out what home remedies will work, but what's more, which remedies they *like*.

So, do the following in order to be one step ahead of your ailments:

1) First get a notebook. This will be used like your own personal scared medicine book. (Yes, you could probably think of yourself as one of those witch doctors...but no skulls please.)

2) Pick out two illnesses from which you suffer more commonly.

3) Research and choose recipes for each remedy for each illness.

4) Make a list of items you don't have and then gather all ingredients.

5) Prepare each remedy.

6) Use your senses to familiarize yourself with each remedy. What does each smell like? Look like? Are they thick or watery? Do you like the taste?

7) Repeat with other remedies you may be interested in testing out. Experiment with different ingredients and even formulate your own secret home remedy specialty.

8) Keep notes of all these things in your notebook.

Grow Your Own Herbs

You can even grow your own herbs at home. The great thing about this is that you will never run out of stocks especially when you need them the most.

- Herb Gardens

Herbs can be grown easily in the backyard, in the smallest available space because most of them have adventitious root which doesn't require a deep rooted seating. You can also grow herbs inside your own home, which is nice when you really want or unexpectedly need them.

- Nursery beds

If you're interested in expanding your herb garden, you may decide to build a nursery bed. A nursery bed is just a larger space in the garden where you can plant your desired herbs.

Some of the plants require that you plant them in special places with special conditions such as lower sunlight and more water (luckily, most herbs grow from stem cutting) because they often cannot withstand the harsh condition of the open field. When the herbs have stayed in the nursery bed for seven to fourteen days, they are transferred to a vessel where they are allowed to grow permanently.

- Nursing your herbs and plants

Nursing your herbs and plants involves watering them once or twice a day, pulling weeds that begin to grow in or around the plants, and when the air is dry, you will need to mulch the soil by covering them with green leaves to reduce water loss. This will keep them growing as needed.

<u>Exercise</u>: If You Build It, It Will Grow

It may not be "Field of Dreams", but having herbs at your fingertips can be done fairly easily by re-using items in your home. Just do the following:

1) Find containers such as cottage cheese or yogurt containers, and poke holes in the bottom. The only requirements are that the containers are at least 2" deep and allow for drainage.

2) Fill the containers with Loam soil, which can be found at any garden center, or stores such as Home Depot or Lowes.

3) If desired, you can also add compost manure generated from your decomposing vegetables at home to add nutrients to the soil.

4) Implant herbs or herb branches into the soil.

5) Be sure to read directions and place herbs in appropriate temperatures and sunlight.

CHAPTER 6

Remedies within the Outdoors

Seek Mother Nature For Help

Now that you have become more familiar with home remedies in an everyday capacity, you can take that knowledge and begin applying it in other areas, such as camping.

They may be called "home remedies," but they can apply elsewhere.

Just as when you are at home, you may find yourself out in the middle of nowhere, caught in a camping trip gone wrong (remember "The Great Outdoors"?) and need quick remedies.

Common problems when camping include the following:

1) Poison Ivy.

2) Annoying critters.

3) Bugs, bugs, and more bugs.

Finding Remedies Around Your Environment

While you may not be Bear Grylls or on an episode of "Survivor" or "Naked and Afraid," Depending on your environment knowing which helpful home remedies to use while camping would be beneficial should you need to find them.

- Know what poison ivy looks like, and what kind of vegetation is found in the area where you will be camping.

- Know home remedies for keeping bugs at bay, or critters away, should you accidentally forget items from home that you needed.

- Know how nature can aid in first aid.

In the old days past, people out in the wild usually fed collected herbs to animals or observed if other animals/insects ate these unknown perennials. If the animals survived, they would know the herbs were safe. Also squeezing the leaves for the fluid to drop on the skin that resulted in an irritation meant a bad sign.

Basically when you're in the wilderness (think alone on an island by yourself with no knowledge of your surrounding) and you life depends on it, you have to be sort of a "MacGuyver."

For example, look out for herbs with sugary contents such as flower nectars. They will be good for wounds because sugar causes coagulation of blood. Cobwebs on leaves can serve as immediate cotton wools to seal off wounds and limit blood loss, which were used hundred years ago to stop bleeding due to their enriched vitamin K property for clotting blood.

Exercise: Create Your Outdoor Remedies

Assume you are camping and have had the following things happen during your trip for which you need a home remedy to solve the problem:

1) Raccoons seem to be taking over your camp and you need a way to not only keep them at bay, but want to make them never come back again…without exterminating them.

2) Your spouse and child went exploring…right in to poison ivy. You forgot the calamine lotion and need to

come up with a new remedy (and no, getting in the car and running to the nearest Walgreens isn't a home remedy...better yet, let's pretend you're all on that deserted island.)

3) You went hiking and upon your return discovered that an animal had gone through all of your food. You need to know what around you in nature can be eaten.

For each of the above scenarios, research and write down 2 or 3 home remedies that could address and resolve the problem.

Don't forget about your personalized home remedies notebook to put all these in for future references.

CHAPTER 7

Integration of Traditional Remedies with Modern Medicines

The Benefits Are Obvious

Having come this far, the benefits of home remedies are glaring. A recap of some of the benefits are as follows.

1) **They save time, and money.** Home remedies are readily available or close at hand. When there is an emergency, there is the desire for urgent relief. Opting for medical attention may cause an unnecessary waste of

time for more common problems. Home remedies in those cases may be an equally *effective*, and more *cost-effective* option.

2) **They have little to no side effects.** Since home remedies are derived from some of the ingredients that form your daily meal and natural products, it is less likely to cause side effects (except if the person is allergic to one of the ingredients, of course.)

3) **They can provide a sense of immediate relief.** There is a sense of relief you feel when the solution to your problem is close at hand and you can address is quickly. That is the kind of calm you will have if you know you can easily dash to the kitchen or backyard and solve the problem.

4) **They are multi-functional.** Most home remedies have broad spectrum of applications. Leaves, for example, will nourish you with the necessary dietary

fiber you need, yet they also supply you with vitamins and other nutrients.

Final Exercise: Become A Home Remedy Guru

Have you observed that some illnesses have similar remedies, and some remedies have similar ingredients? Well, you're not imagining it, they do.

Let's prove it by doing the following:

1) Make a set diagram of two circles intercepting to form another smaller circle between them.

2) In the areas of each of the two big circles, write the name of the two illnesses for which you've noticed there may be a common remedy.

3) In the smaller circle in the middle, write the ingredients that is common to them.

Do you notice it becoming easier to remember what functions different foods, herbs, spices, etc., serve because of the mutual remedies they provide?

Forget the gap, find where they overlap.

Again to be a broken record, pull out your handy-dandy medicine man/woman's notebook guide to jot your findings.

Final Thoughts

Home remedies should form an essential part of every person's quick solution guide. Besides the use of home remedies to cure illnesses or combat health challenges, some of the edible remedies often add nutritional supplements that may be lacking in your daily diet.

There are phytochemicals inherent in green leaves that are very effective in mopping up the free radicals from the blood which when left unchecked, may result in serious health challenges.

Another problem with the conventional drugs is that of overdose. There have been reported cases of parents leaving their children at home and the children, in their parent's absence, got ahold of pills and swallowed them to their detriment.

A report from the Foundation for A Drug Free World shows that every day in the US, 2,500 youths ages 12 to 17 abuse a prescription pain reliever for the first time. This is disastrous to our society. If this trend continues unabated, what kind of leaders do we hope to have tomorrow?

The bottom line is that homeopathic remedies pose less danger because rarely can they be abused nor do they normally have an overdose. And, they don't require a medical degree to dispense.

If you followed this training from the beginning, you should be well on your way to becoming a home remedy expert.

Now You Know!

We have now gone from - *NOT knowing*...to *KNOWING*.

Doesn't it feel great? As cliché as the proverbial saying goes: knowledge is, indeed, power. The more you know, the more empowered you become. Not knowing is defeating, as you succumb to feelings of helplessness and surrendering of your own self.

Of course, acquiring knowledge is a never-ending quest. There is a great saying by Nobel Prize French author Andre Gide: "Believe those who are seeking the truth. Doubt those who find it."

At the very least, we hope we have set you off in the right path in regards to what you have set out to know, and that you have enjoyed our little journey together for the time you have spent with us.

If you can tell us how we did, that would be very appreciated! We value your feedback and always look forward to hearing from you, or if there is any way we could improve the entire experience for you. If you have a success story, even better - please let us know!

http://www.KnowItExpress.com

Don't forget to stay in contact for we would love to connect with you.

https://www.facebook.com/KnowItExpress
https://twitter.com/KnowItExpress
https://plus.google.com/+KnowItExpress

What would you like to know? Let us know!

CONTACT US

Now onward for more power to you, and thank you!

Home Remedies Express